Dedicated to Dr. Uzodinma Raphael Dim, a transformative mentor who enlightened me about the workings of the world, reshaping my mindset along the way.

Mechanisms of cardiac arrhythmias

Imagine a symphony of the human body, where the heart serves as the conductor, orchestrating the rhythmic dance of life. However, within this intricate composition, there exists a fascinating and captivating phenomenon known as cardiac arrhythmias. These enigmatic disturbances in the heart's rhythm possess an undeniable allure, presenting clinicians with a captivating challenge and holding the potential to profoundly impact the health and well-being of our patients.

Cardiac arrhythmias, like elusive musical notes that stray from the expected melody, disrupt the harmonious beat of the heart. They come in various forms, each with its unique cadence, from the sporadic skipping of beats to the rapid, chaotic whirlwind that threatens the stability of the entire symphony. These irregularities can occur in people of all ages, from the young to the elderly, and can arise from a multitude of causes, both congenital and acquired.

What makes cardiac arrhythmias so intriguing is their ability to manifest silently, lurking beneath the surface, undetected until they reveal themselves in unexpected and potentially life-threatening ways. They challenge our understanding of the heart's intricate electrical system, forcing us to delve into the depths of its mysteries to unravel the mechanisms behind its emergence.

The pursuit of deciphering these arrhythmic puzzles has led to remarkable advances in medical technology and therapies. From the development of high-resolution imaging techniques and wearable devices that can monitor heart rhythms in real time to the creation of sophisticated algorithms and artificial intelligence systems that aid in diagnosis and treatment, the field of cardiac electrophysiology has become a captivating blend of science and innovation.

Moreover, the impact of cardiac arrhythmias reaches far beyond the individual patient. It reverberates through the corridors of healthcare, inspiring collaboration among medical professionals, researchers, and engineers to push the boundaries of knowledge and devise novel ways to restore the symphony of the heart. It has sparked a collective quest to develop safer and more effective treatments, such as catheter-based ablation techniques and implantable devices that can modulate the heart's electrical activity, offering hope to countless individuals affected by these rhythmic disturbances.

Cardiac arrhythmias, with their intricate complexities and potential consequences, beckon us to explore the delicate balance between the rhythms of life and the symphony of the heart. Understanding their nuances and unraveling their secrets holds the promise of improving patient outcomes, enhancing quality of life, and shaping the future of cardiovascular medicine. In this captivating journey, clinicians and researchers alike are united by a shared fascination—an unwavering determination to decode the enigma of cardiac arrhythmias and compose a harmonious melody of health and vitality for all.0

Cardiac physiology

At the core of this magnificent organ lies a captivating arrangement of four chambers, each with its own vital role. The right and left atria serve as receiving chambers, welcoming deoxygenated and oxygenated blood, respectively. The right atrium receives deoxygenated blood from the superior vena cava, while the left atrium receives freshly oxygenated blood from the pulmonary veins.

As blood enters the heart, it encounters a series of critical valves that ensure unidirectional flow. The tricuspid valve, situated between the right atrium and right ventricle, acts as a gateway, permitting blood to pass through while preventing backflow. Similarly, the mitral valve (also known as the bicuspid valve) orchestrates the flow between the left atrium and left ventricle.

Now, let us delve deeper into the heart's chambers. The right ventricle, powered by the forceful contraction of its muscular walls, propels deoxygenated blood forward. This blood exits the heart through the pulmonary valve, embarking on a journey through the pulmonary trunk and pulmonary arteries. Within the lungs, a marvelous exchange occurs, with carbon dioxide being expelled and oxygen infusing the blood, transforming it into a revitalizing elixir.

Reinvigorated by oxygen, the blood rejoins the symphony of circulation, returning to the heart via the pulmonary veins. The left atrium, acting as a gracious host, welcomes this oxygen-rich blood. It then elegantly guides it through the mitral valve, allowing entry into the left ventricle.

The left ventricle, the powerhouse of the heart, contracts forcefully, generating the necessary pressure to propel oxygenated blood forward. Through the aortic valve, the blood departs the heart, embarking on a grand expedition through the aorta—the largest artery in the body. From there, it branches into an intricate network of arteries, delivering precious oxygen to every nook and cranny of our being.

Understanding this captivating anatomy is crucial in comprehending the mechanisms underlying arrhythmias. By grasping the interplay of the heart's chambers, valves, veins, and arteries, we gain a comprehensive foundation for effective diagnosis, education, and management of these rhythm disturbances. It empowers healthcare professionals to navigate the complexities of arrhythmias, guiding interventions and treatments that can restore the heart's harmonious symphony, ensuring optimal health and vitality for individuals affected by these conditions.

The conduction system

The cardiac electrical system refers to the specialized network of cells that generate and conduct electrical impulses throughout the heart, regulating its rhythm and coordinating its contractions. The main components of the cardiac electrical system include the sinoatrial node (SA node), atrioventricular node (AV node), and the bundle of His, and Purkinje fibers.

Within the intricate landscape of cardiac physiology, the conduction system of the heart orchestrates a symphony of electrical impulses, ensuring the coordinated and efficient pumping of blood. Understanding this intricate network is essential for comprehending the development of arrhythmias and devising appropriate interventions.

At the heart's epicenter lies the sinoatrial (SA) node, a specialized cluster of cells located in the right atrium. The SA node acts as the natural pacemaker, generating electrical signals that initiate each heartbeat. From this remarkable node, the electrical impulses propagate through the atria, stimulating their contraction.

The journey of these electrical impulses continues as they traverse the atrioventricular (AV) node, strategically positioned between the atria and ventricles. The AV node serves as a crucial bridge, momentarily delaying the electrical signal. This delay allows the atria to fully contract, ensuring optimal blood filling within the ventricles before the ventricular contraction commences. This synchronized timing optimizes the efficiency of blood flow and prevents rapid or irregular heart rhythms.

Once the electrical impulses traverse the AV node, they travel through a specialized pathway known as the bundle of His. This bundle of conducting fibers efficiently conducts the electrical signals from the AV node down into the ventricles. As the bundle of His descends, it branches into the left and right bundle branches, extending into their respective ventricles.

The final stage of this remarkable journey involves the rapid dissemination of electrical impulses through a network of specialized fibers called the Purkinje fibers. These fibers form an intricate web throughout the ventricles, ensuring rapid and synchronized contraction of the ventricular muscle fibers. This coordinated contraction effectively pumps blood out of the heart and into the circulatory system, supplying vital oxygen and nutrients to the body's organs and tissues.

The harmonious interplay between the SA node, AV node, bundle of His, and Purkinje fibers is crucial for maintaining the synchronized contraction of the atria and ventricles. This synchronized rhythm ensures efficient blood circulation and optimal cardiac function. Disruptions or abnormalities within this intricate conduction system can lead to arrhythmias, compromising the heart's ability to pump effectively.

By comprehending the elegant sequence of electrical impulses generated by the SA node and conducted through the AV node, the bundle of His, and Purkinje fibers, healthcare professionals gain valuable insights into the origins and mechanisms of arrhythmias. This knowledge forms the foundation for accurate diagnosis, appropriate management, and the development of targeted interventions aimed at restoring the heart's electrical harmony and preserving cardiovascular health.

Legend
SA 60-100
AV 40-60
Purkinje fibers 20-40

Brady <60
Tachy>100

What is an arrhythmia?

In the captivating realm of cardiac health, arrhythmias emerge as intriguing phenomena characterized by irregularities in the heart's rhythm. These irregular heart rhythms manifest when the normally generated electrical impulses from the sinoatrial (SA) node deviate from their expected patterns. Arrhythmias present themselves in various forms, with four prominent classifications that capture our attention: Bradycardia, Tachycardia, Atrial Fibrillation (AFib), and Ventricular Fibrillation (VFib). Each classification represents a distinct pattern of irregularity, signifying a specific disruption in the heart's rhythmic function. Therefore, the diagnosis and treatment of arrhythmias necessitate a personalized and meticulous approach, tailored to the unique characteristics of each individual's condition.

What can increase the risk of developing an arrhythmia

-Heart diseases

1. Coronary Artery Disease (CAD) is a pathological condition characterized by the accumulation of plaque, leading to the narrowing or occlusion of arteries responsible for delivering blood to the heart. This atherosclerotic process comprises the blood flow to the cardiac muscle, resulting in inadequate oxygen supply. Consequently, this oxygen deprivation can precipitate the occurrence of arrhythmias, denoting irregular electrical activity within the myocardium.

2. Heart failure; Characterized by the heart's diminished capacity to pump blood efficiently. The cardiac electrical system may change when the myocardium deteriorates, increasing the risk of arrhythmias in our patients. Arrhythmias may also develop as a result of the buildup of fluid in the lungs and other tissues, a typical side effect of heart failure.

-Cardiomyopathy

1. Often observed in electrical remodeling, cardiomyopathy can change the electrical makeup of the heart. The structural flaws and scarring of the myocardium may obstruct the heart's normal conduction pathways, leading to abnormal electrical impulses and arrhythmias.

2. Ischemia, which refers to inadequate blood supply to a specific organ or tissue, can lead to the development of arrhythmias in the context of cardiomyopathy. This supply can cause an imbalance in the concentration of ions (such as potassium, sodium, and calcium) within the heart cells, leading to changes in the electrical activity and rhythm of the heart.

-Imbalances in electrolyte levels

1. Hypokalemia: Low potassium levels can impair the repolarization phase of the cardiac cells, delaying the recovery time for electrical activity.
2. - Hypernatremia: Elevated sodium levels can cause an increase in the action potential duration, potentially leading to arrhythmias, especially in individuals with existing heart conditions.
3. - Hyponatremia: Low sodium levels can result in changes to the action potential configuration, leading to a prolonged QT interval and an increased risk of arrhythmias.
4. - Hypocalcemia: Decreased calcium levels can impair the conduction of electrical impulses and cause abnormalities in the repolarization phase, leading to arrhythmias.
5. - Hypomagnesemia: Low magnesium levels can increase the risk of ventricular arrhythmias, particularly in the presence of other electrolyte imbalances.

-COVID-19

1. COVID-19 triggers an immune response, and in severe cases, it can lead to an excessive and uncontrolled inflammatory response known as a cytokine storm. Inflammation and cytokine release can affect the heart's electrical stability and increase the risk of arrhythmias. A cytokine storm refers to an overactive immune response resulting in the excessive release of cytokines. (small proteins vital for cell signaling) This overdrive can lead to widespread inflammation, causing symptoms like fever, fatigue, shortness of breath, and in

extreme cases, organ failure. Cytokine storms can occur due to infection, autoimmune diseases, certain cancers, and severe cases of COVID-19. Although there's no direct link between cytokine storms and arrhythmias, severe cases of certain diseases, like COVID-19, can lead to a cytokine storm causing multisystem organ failure, including heart failure, which can indirectly trigger arrhythmias. Moreover, inflammation due to a cytokine storm may increase arrhythmia risk.

Assessments and Measures

Diagnosing and assessing arrhythmia severity, including bradycardia, tachycardia, atrial fibrillation (AFib), and ventricular fibrillation (V-Fib), requires a series of tests:

1. Electrocardiogram (ECG): A primary tool to record the heart's electrical activity and identify arrhythmias.

2. Holter Monitor: A portable device to monitor heart rhythms during regular activities, useful for detecting arrhythmias not evident in a standard ECG.

3. Stress Test: This test checks if physical exercise triggers an arrhythmia.

4. Echocardiogram: A non-invasive imaging technique used to identify underlying conditions potentially causing an arrhythmia.

5. Cardiac Catheterization and Electrophysiology (EP) Study: Invasive tests that allow direct recording of the heart's electrical activity to pinpoint the arrhythmia source.

6. Blood Tests: Used to identify underlying conditions like thyroid disorders or electrolyte imbalances that may contribute to the arrhythmia.

   1. Complete blood count (CBC): A CBC measures various components of the blood, including red blood cells, white blood cells, and platelets. Certain blood disorders or infections can indirectly affect the heart and potentially contribute to arrhythmias.

   2. Cardiac biomarkers: Blood tests can measure specific substances released into the bloodstream during heart muscle damage or stress. Elevated levels of cardiac biomarkers, such as troponin or creatine kinase-MB (CK-MB), may indicate a

heart attack or other cardiac conditions that can cause arrhythmias.

3. Thyroid function tests: Thyroid hormone imbalances, such as hyperthyroidism or hypothyroidism, can affect the heart rhythm and lead to arrhythmias

4. Electrolyte levels: Imbalances in electrolytes such as potassium, calcium, and magnesium can affect the heart's electrical conduction system and potentially contribute to arrhythmias

These assessments provide comprehensive information to diagnose the arrhythmia type, determine its severity, and guide the appropriate treatment plan.

Mapping the Electrical Symphony: A Journey into EKG Lead Placement and Interpretation

The electrocardiogram (EKG) is the symphony of the heart's electrical activity, a complex melody that requires precise mapping. EKG lead placement and interpretation are essential components of this intricate process, guiding healthcare professionals to diagnose and treat a wide range of cardiac conditions. In this journey, we will explore the art of EKG lead placement and interpretation, unravel the mystery of unipolar and bipolar leads, and discover how to identify the elusive sinus rhythm.

EKG Lead Placement:

EKG lead placement is the process of positioning the electrodes, or leads, on the patient's chest, arms, and legs, allowing for the capture of the heart's electrical activity. The standard ECG consists of 12 leads, each with a unique perspective on the heart's electrical activity. The placement of these leads forms a pattern that healthcare professionals use to diagnose and monitor cardiac conditions.

The V1 and V2 leads are positioned on the right side of the chest, while the V3 to V6 leads are placed on the left side. The limb leads, consisting of the I, II, III, aVR, aVL, and aVF leads, are positioned on the arms and legs. The precise positioning of the leads is crucial, as it affects the accuracy of the EKG readings.

Unipolar and Bipolar Leads:

EKG leads are classified into two categories: unipolar and bipolar. Unipolar leads record the heart's electrical activity from a single electrode, while bipolar leads record the electrical activity between two electrodes. The standard ECG uses both types of leads, with the limb leads being bipolar and the chest leads being unipolar.

The unipolar leads, V1 to V6, record the electrical activity of the heart in a specific direction, with each lead having its unique view. The bipolar leads, I, II, and III record the electrical activity between two electrodes, providing a different perspective on the heart's electrical activity.

Sinus Rhythm Interpretation:

Sinus rhythm is the normal electrical activity of the heart, where the electrical impulses originate from the sinus node, the heart's natural pacemaker. It is essential to identify sinus rhythm on an EKG, as it serves as a baseline for diagnosing and monitoring cardiac conditions.

To identify sinus rhythm, healthcare professionals look for specific characteristics on the EKG. The P wave, representing atrial depolarization, should have a consistent shape and duration. The QRS complex, representing ventricular depolarization, should have a consistent shape and duration as well. Additionally, the heart rate should fall within a normal range of 60 to 100 beats per minute.

Conclusion:

EKG lead placement and interpretation are essential components of diagnosing and monitoring cardiac conditions. Precise placement of the leads and accurate interpretation of the electrical activity of the heart are crucial in identifying sinus rhythm and detecting any abnormalities. By understanding the intricacies of EKG lead placement and interpretation, healthcare professionals can provide the best possible care for their patient's cardiac health.

Unveiling the Intriguing PQRST Wave and EKGs

Welcome to the captivating world of the PQRST wave and EKGs! In this short page, we will explore the fascinating connection between these two concepts.

1. The PQRST Wave:

The PQRST wave represents the electrical activity of the heart during a cardiac cycle. It consists of the P-wave, QRS complex, and T-wave. The P-wave indicates atrial contraction, the QRS complex reflects ventricular contraction, and the T-wave represents ventricular relaxation.

2. Electrocardiography (EKG):

EKG is a non-invasive test that records the heart's electrical activity. It involves placing electrodes on the skin, which detect and amplify signals. The resulting waveform provides valuable information about heart rhythm, rate, and health.

3. Clinical Applications:

PQRST and EKGs have various clinical applications:

- Diagnosing Cardiac Disorders: Analyzing the PQRST wave on an EKG helps identify irregular heart rhythms and conditions like atrial fibrillation and ventricular tachycardia.

- Evaluating Heart Health: EKGs assess heart size, structure, and blood supply. They aid in detecting heart diseases such as coronary artery disease and heart attacks.

- Monitoring Treatment Progress: EKGs track the effects of medications, interventions, or surgeries on the heart, helping healthcare professionals make informed decisions.

Unveiling the Mystery of the Short PR Interval: Unraveling its Impact and Innovative Solutions

Step into the fascinating world of electrocardiograms (ECGs) and discover the enigmatic realm of the PR interval. Deep within the intricate workings of our hearts, lies a curious anomaly known as the short PR interval. Buckle up as we embark on an exhilarating journey to unravel its impact and explore the cutting-edge solutions that hold the key to managing this captivating condition.

In the context of cardiac electrophysiology, the term "short PR interval" refers to a measurement of time on an electrocardiogram (ECG).

It specifically represents the duration between two specific points on the ECG waveform.

To understand the concept of an interval, it's important to know that an ECG is a graphical representation of the electrical activity of the heart. It displays the changes in electrical potential as the heart goes through its rhythmical contractions.

The PR interval, in particular, measures the time it takes for the electrical signal to travel from the atria (the upper chambers of the heart) to the ventricles (the lower chambers of the heart) through the atrioventricular (AV) node, which acts as a gatekeeper for the electrical impulses.

A short PR interval means that the time it takes for the electrical signal to travel through the AV node and reach the ventricles is shorter than what is considered normal. It indicates a rapid conduction of electrical impulses from the atria to the ventricles.

The duration of the PR interval is measured in milliseconds (ms) on the ECG. Normal PR intervals typically range between 120 and 200 ms. If the PR interval is shorter than this range, it is considered a short PR interval.

The significance of a short PR interval depends on the context and the individual's overall heart health. In some cases, a short PR interval may be benign and not cause any health concerns. However, in other situations, it can be associated with certain cardiac conditions or abnormalities, such as pre-excitation syndromes like Wolff-Parkinson-White (WPW) syndrome.

In summary, the term "short PR interval" refers to a measurement of time on an ECG that represents the duration between two specific points on the waveform. It indicates a rapid conduction of electrical impulses from the atria to the ventricles. The significance of a short PR interval depends on various factors and may require further evaluation to determine its implications for a specific individual.

Complications:

1. Arrhythmias: A short PR interval can predispose individuals to certain arrhythmias, such as supraventricular tachycardia (SVT) or atrial fibrillation. These irregular heart rhythms can cause symptoms like palpitations, dizziness, or fainting.

2. Risk of sudden cardiac arrest: In some cases, a short PR interval may be associated with conditions like Wolff-Parkinson-White (WPW) syndrome, which can increase the risk of potentially life-threatening arrhythmias and sudden cardiac arrest.

3. Hemodynamic instability: In situations where the rapid conduction of electrical impulses leads to an abnormal heart rhythm, it can compromise effective blood pumping and lead to hemodynamic instability.

Solutions:

1. Medications: Depending on the specific arrhythmia or underlying condition, medications may be prescribed to regulate heart rhythm and prevent arrhythmias. Antiarrhythmic medications or beta-blockers are commonly used in such cases.

2. Catheter ablation: In some cases of arrhythmias associated with a short PR interval, a procedure called catheter ablation may be recommended. This involves using catheters to deliver energy (such as radiofrequency or cryotherapy) to specific areas of the heart to disrupt the abnormal electrical pathways causing the arrhythmia.

3. Implantable devices: For individuals at a high risk of sudden cardiac arrest, the implantation of an implantable cardioverter-defibrillator (ICD) may be considered. An ICD continuously monitors the heart's rhythm and delivers an electrical shock to restore normal rhythm if a dangerous arrhythmia occurs.

4. Lifestyle modifications: Certain lifestyle changes can help manage and reduce the risk of arrhythmias. These may include avoiding triggers like excessive caffeine or alcohol, managing stress levels, maintaining a healthy weight, and engaging in regular physical activity.

5. Regular monitoring and follow-up: Individuals with a short PR interval or associated conditions may require regular monitoring by a cardiologist to assess heart rhythm, adjust medications if necessary, and ensure optimal management.

Harmonies of the Heart: Unveiling the Enigmatic Symphony of ST Elevation and ST Depression

Welcome to the melodious world of ST elevation and ST depression, where the heart's symphony unfolds on the grand stage of an electrocardiogram (ECG). Just as a conductor directs an orchestra, the ECG reveals the intricate electrical movements within our hearts. Let us dive into this harmonious journey and explore the contrasting melodies of ST elevation and ST depression.

Imagine a crescendo of electrical activity as the heart enters the ST segment, the tranquil interval between ventricular depolarization and repolarization. Normally, this segment lies peacefully along the baseline, like a calm river flowing gently. However, when the heart experiences an electrical aberration, the symphony takes an unexpected turn.

ST elevation, the rising cadence of the heart's melody, signifies a moment of distress. It is often associated with an acute myocardial infarction, where a coronary artery becomes blocked, thwarting the life-giving flow of blood to a portion of the heart muscle. This interruption causes ischemia, akin to a sudden silence in the symphony, followed by a powerful surge of electrical activity that elevates the ST segment. Like a conductor raising their baton, the ECG reveals this dramatic elevation, alerting clinicians to the urgent need for intervention.

Yet, the orchestra of the heart holds more than one captivating tune. ST depression, a somber descent in the ECG's melodic notes, tells a different tale. It is the subtle whisper of ischemia, a gentle plea for attention. Picture an orchestra playing softly, the violins delicately weeping, as the heart encounters reduced blood flow and oxygen supply. This condition often arises from coronary artery disease, where plaques obstruct the coronary arteries, limiting the heart's nourishment. In response, the ST segment descends, mirroring the melancholy of the heart's struggle.

During an exercise stress test, the symphony reaches its climax. The heart is challenged like a virtuoso performer pushed to their limits. As the body demands increased oxygen and energy, the ECG becomes a conductor's baton, guiding us through the heart's response. Should ST depression emerge during this strenuous performance, it hints at significant coronary artery disease, cautioning us to heed the call for further investigation.

Beyond the grand melodies of acute myocardial infarction and coronary artery disease, other conditions add their unique harmonies to the ECG score. Pericarditis and myocarditis, the fiery dances of inflammation, may also raise the ST segment, but with their distinct rhythms and patterns. Rare genetic conditions like Brugada syndrome and early repolarization syndrome introduce their compositions, painting a symphony of complexity that astounds both musician and listener.

In this mesmerizing symphony of ST elevation and ST depression, the heart's electrical tale unfolds. Each note, each rise and fall, carries a story of its own—a story that guides clinicians in their quest to heal and restore the heart's rhythm. So let us listen attentively to the ECG's melody, appreciating the cadences of ST elevation and ST depression, as they reveal the secrets of the heart's symphony.

The Elusive Long QT Interval: Unveiling its Impact on the Heart

Hidden within the intricate pattern of an electrocardiogram (ECG) lies a fascinating phenomenon known as the long QT interval. This seemingly innocuous prolongation of the QT interval, representing the electrical depolarization and repolarization of the heart, can have profound implications for cardiac health. In this captivating journey, we will explore the captivating effects of a long QT interval on the heart and its potential consequences.

I. Unraveling the Long QT Interval:

1. The QT Interval Enigma: The QT interval represents the time duration of ventricular depolarization and repolarization on an ECG. When this interval is prolonged, exceeding normal limits (typically >440 milliseconds in males and >460 milliseconds in females), it is referred to as a long QT interval.

2. The Impact on Repolarization: A prolonged QT interval indicates delayed ventricular repolarization, specifically the time it takes for the heart muscle to reset electrically between beats. This delay can disrupt the heart's electrical stability and increase the risk of arrhythmias.

II. The Dance of Arrhythmias:

1. Torsades de Pointes (TdP): The most notable consequence of a prolonged QT interval is an increased susceptibility to a specific type of ventricular arrhythmia called Torsades de Pointes. This mesmerizing arrhythmia is characterized by a twisting or spiraling pattern of the heart rhythm on the ECG, leading to rapid and irregular heartbeats. TdP can cause palpitations, dizziness, syncope (fainting), and, in severe cases, life-threatening ventricular fibrillation and sudden cardiac arrest.

2. Ventricular Fibrillation: In some instances, a prolonged QT interval can trigger ventricular fibrillation, a chaotic and uncoordinated quivering of the ventricles. This condition disrupts the heart's ability to pump blood effectively and can rapidly progress to cardiac arrest if not treated promptly.

III. Unveiling the Culprits:

1. Inherited Long QT Syndrome (LQTS): A significant number of cases with a prolonged QT interval are due to an inherited condition known as Long QT Syndrome. This syndrome is caused by genetic mutations affecting the ion channels responsible for the heart's electrical activity, leading to delayed repolarization. Several subtypes of LQTS exist, each associated with specific genetic abnormalities and varying risks of arrhythmias.

2. Acquired Causes: Prolonged QT intervals can also result from certain medications (e.g., some antiarrhythmics, antibiotics, antipsychotics), electrolyte imbalances (e.g., low potassium or magnesium levels), medical conditions (e.g., heart disease, thyroid disorders), or even illicit drug use.

IV. Seeking Solutions:

1. Risk Stratification: Identifying individuals with a prolonged QT interval and determining their risk of arrhythmias is crucial. This involves a comprehensive evaluation, including a thorough medical history, ECG analysis, genetic testing (in cases of suspected inherited LQTS), and assessment of any underlying medical conditions or medications.

Junctional rhythm,

Known as nodal rhythm, is a type of cardiac arrhythmia characterized by the abnormal initiation of electrical impulses within the atrioventricular (AV) junction of the heart. In this rhythm, the AV node or the surrounding tissues take over the role of the heart's natural pacemaker, the sinoatrial (SA) node, which is responsible for initiating the electrical signals that regulate the heart's contractions.

Normally, the SA node generates electrical impulses that travel through the atria, causing them to contract and pump blood into the ventricles. The impulses then pass through the AV node and into the ventricles, causing them to contract and pump blood to the rest of the body. However, in a junctional rhythm, the AV node becomes the dominant pacemaker, generating its electrical signals and initiating the heartbeats independent of the SA node.

There are several possible reasons why a junctional rhythm may occur. It can be a compensatory response when the SA node is not functioning properly or is unable to generate electrical impulses at a normal rate. It can also arise as a result of certain medications, electrolyte imbalances, heart disease, or after cardiac surgery.

Clinically, junctional rhythm can present with a variety of symptoms or it may be asymptomatic. Common symptoms include palpitations, dizziness, lightheadedness, fatigue, and shortness of breath. The severity of symptoms can vary depending on the underlying cause, the rate of the rhythm, and the overall health of the individual.

On an electrocardiogram (ECG), junctional rhythm is characterized by specific patterns. The P wave, which represents atrial depolarization, may be absent or may appear inverted or after the QRS complex. The QRS complex, which represents ventricular depolarization, is typically normal in shape and duration. The heart rate in junctional rhythm can range from 40 to 60 beats per minute, although it can be faster or slower depending on the specific circumstances.

The management of junctional rhythm depends on several factors, including the underlying cause, the presence of symptoms, and the hemodynamic stability of the patient. In some cases, no treatment may be necessary if the rhythm is transient or benign. However, if symptoms are present or if the rhythm persists and causes hemodynamic instability, intervention may be required.

Treatment options for junctional rhythm may include addressing the underlying cause, such as correcting electrolyte imbalances or adjusting medications. In cases where the rhythm is persistent and symptomatic, medications such as beta-blockers or calcium channel blockers may be prescribed to slow the heart rate and restore normal rhythm. In severe cases or when other treatment measures are ineffective, invasive procedures such as catheter ablation or pacemaker implantation may be considered.

In conclusion, junctional rhythm is an abnormal cardiac arrhythmia characterized by the abnormal initiation of electrical impulses within the AV junction of the heart. It can occur due to various factors and may present with a range of symptoms. The management of junctional rhythm depends on the underlying cause and the severity of symptoms, with treatment options ranging from conservative measures to invasive procedures. Proper diagnosis, evaluation, and individualized treatment plans are essential in effectively managing junctional rhythm and ensuring optimal cardiac function.

Bradycardia; the slow beat

Bradycardia is characterized by an abnormally slow heart rate. In our patients with bradycardia, the heart beats slower than the normal resting heart rate, which is typically between 60 and 100 beats per minute in adults. Bradycardia can result from various factors, including age, certain medications, heart conditions, underlying health issues, or an imbalance in the electrical signals that regulate the heart's rhythm. Symptoms of bradycardia may include fatigue, dizziness, lightheadedness, fainting, shortness of breath, and chest pain.

Bradycardia is a medical condition characterized by an abnormally slow heart rate. While bradycardia itself is a clinical term used to describe a heart rate below 60 beats per minute, it is important to understand various real-life examples and scenarios where bradycardia may occur.

1. Athletes and Physically Fit Individuals:

One common example of bradycardia is seen in highly trained athletes or individuals who engage in regular intense physical activity. Their bodies adapt to the increased demand for oxygen and improved cardiovascular efficiency. As a result, their resting heart rates can be significantly lower than the average population, often ranging from 40 to 60 beats per minute.

For instance, professional endurance athletes like long-distance runners or cyclists may have resting heart rates as low as 40 beats per minute due to their well-conditioned cardiovascular systems. This lower heart rate allows their hearts to pump efficiently and deliver oxygen to the muscles during exercise.

2. Aging Population:

Another real-life example of bradycardia is associated with the aging process. As people get older, changes occur in the electrical system of the heart, which can cause a naturally slower heart rate. This age-related bradycardia is typically benign and not a cause for concern unless it leads to symptoms or complications.

3. Medications:

Certain medications, especially those used to manage heart conditions, can cause bradycardia as a side effect. For instance, beta-blockers, commonly prescribed for hypertension or heart disease, work by slowing down the heart rate and reducing the force of contraction. While this can be beneficial in certain cases, it may result in bradycardia as an unintended consequence.

4. Underlying Medical Conditions:

Bradycardia can also be a symptom or result of underlying medical conditions. For example, individuals with hypothyroidism, a condition where the thyroid gland doesn't produce enough thyroid hormone, may experience bradycardia due to the hormone's role in regulating heart rate. Similarly, heart diseases such as heart block, myocarditis, or coronary artery disease can interfere with the heart's electrical signals, leading to a slower heart rate.

5. Vagal Stimulation:

The vagus nerve, which plays a vital role in regulating heart rate, can be stimulated in certain situations, causing bradycardia. This can occur during activities such as straining during bowel movements, coughing forcefully, or bearing down while lifting heavy weights. These actions can activate the vagus nerve, resulting in a temporary slowing of the heart rate.

racing heart: tachycardia

Tachycardia is a common cardiac condition characterized by an abnormally rapid heart rate. This page aims to provide a comprehensive overview of tachycardia, including its causes, symptoms, diagnosis, and management strategies. By exploring the complexities of this condition, we can better understand its impact on individuals' lives and the importance of effective treatment.

Definition and Mechanism:

Tachycardia refers to a heart rate that exceeds the normal resting rate. It is typically defined as a heart rate of over 100 beats per minute. Tachycardia can arise from various causes and can affect the heart's electrical system, leading to rapid and irregular heart rhythms.

Causes and Types:

Tachycardia can be caused by multiple factors, including physical exertion, emotional stress, medical conditions, and medication side effects. It can manifest in different forms, including sinus tachycardia, supraventricular tachycardia (SVT), ventricular tachycardia (VT), and atrial fibrillation.

Symptoms and Diagnosis:

The symptoms experienced in tachycardia can vary depending on the underlying cause and individual factors. Common symptoms include rapid heartbeat, palpitations, shortness of breath, dizziness, chest discomfort, and fainting. Diagnosis is typically made through a combination of medical history assessment, physical examination, electrocardiogram (ECG), and additional cardiac tests if needed.

Real-Life Example 1: Sarah's Experience

Sarah, a 30-year-old woman, started noticing episodes of rapid heartbeat accompanied by dizziness and shortness of breath during her daily activities. Concerned, she sought medical attention and was diagnosed with supraventricular tachycardia (SVT). Sarah's healthcare provider prescribed medication to control her heart rate and referred her for further evaluation. Sarah's case illustrates the impact of tachycardia on a person's daily life and emphasizes the importance of seeking medical advice for proper diagnosis and management.

Treatment and Management:

The management of tachycardia aims to control the heart rate, restore normal rhythm, and address any underlying causes or triggers. Treatment options may include lifestyle modifications, medication, electrical cardioversion, catheter ablation, or implantable devices like pacemakers or implantable cardioverter-defibrillators (ICDs). The specific treatment plan will depend on the type of tachycardia, its severity, and individual patient factors.

Real-Life Example 2: John's Treatment Journey

John, a 45-year-old man, was diagnosed with ventricular tachycardia (VT) after experiencing recurrent episodes of rapid heartbeat and lightheadedness. His healthcare provider recommended catheter ablation as a treatment option. John underwent the procedure, which successfully eliminated the abnormal electrical pathways causing his tachycardia. Following the intervention, John's symptoms significantly improved, highlighting the effectiveness of targeted interventions for specific types of tachycardia.

Lifestyle Modifications:

In addition to medical treatments, lifestyle modifications can play a crucial role in managing tachycardia. These may include stress reduction techniques, regular exercise, maintaining a healthy weight, limiting stimulants like caffeine and nicotine, and managing underlying medical conditions such as hypertension or thyroid disorders

Tachy-Brady syndrome,

also known as bradycardia-tachycardia syndrome, is a cardiac condition characterized by alternating episodes of rapid heart rate (tachycardia) followed by abnormally slow heart rate (bradycardia). This condition disrupts the normal rhythm of the heart and can have significant effects on an individual's health. To understand tachy-brady syndrome, it is important to explore its effects, causes, and real-life examples.

Effects of Tachy-Brady Syndrome:
Tachy-brady syndrome can lead to a range of symptoms and complications, depending on the severity and frequency of the abnormal heart rhythms. Some common effects include:

1. Palpitations: Rapid heart rates during tachycardia episodes can cause palpitations, which are sensations of a pounding or irregular heartbeat.

2. Dizziness and Fainting: Abrupt changes in heart rate from tachycardia to bradycardia can result in dizziness, lightheadedness, or even fainting (syncope). These symptoms occur due to inadequate blood flow and reduced oxygen supply to the brain.

3. Fatigue and Weakness: The irregular heart rhythms in tachy-brady syndrome can reduce the heart's efficiency in pumping blood, leading to reduced oxygen supply to the body's tissues. This can result in fatigue, weakness, and reduced exercise tolerance.

4. Heart Failure: In severe cases, tachy-brady syndrome can contribute to the development or worsening of heart failure. The irregular heart rhythms and inefficient pumping of blood can strain the heart over time, leading to symptoms such as shortness of breath, fluid retention, and swelling.

5. Stroke: Tachy-brady syndrome increases the risk of blood clots forming in the heart. If a clot dislodges and travels to the brain, it can cause a stroke, which may result in neurological deficits or even be life-threatening.

Causes of Tachy-Brady Syndrome:
Tachy-Brady syndrome can have various underlying causes, including:

1. Aging: As individuals get older, the electrical system of the heart may change, making them more susceptible to irregular heart rhythms.

2. Underlying Heart Conditions: Structural heart diseases, such as coronary artery disease, heart valve abnormalities, or cardiomyopathy, can disrupt the heart's electrical signals and contribute to tachy-brady syndrome.

3. Medications or Drug Use: Certain medications, such as beta-blockers or antiarrhythmic drugs, may inadvertently contribute to the development of tachy-brady syndrome. Illicit drug use, particularly stimulants, can also disrupt the heart's electrical activity and lead to abnormal heart rhythms.

Real-Life Examples:

Real-life examples of tachy-brady syndrome can vary depending on individual cases and underlying causes. Here are a few examples:

1. Age-Related Tachy-Brady Syndrome: An elderly individual may experience episodes of rapid heart rate (tachycardia) followed by periods of slow heart rate (bradycardia) due to natural changes in the heart's electrical system associated with aging.

2. Structural Heart Disease: A person with underlying heart conditions, such as coronary artery disease or mitral valve prolapse, may develop tachy-brady syndrome due to the abnormal electrical signals caused by these conditions.

3. Medication-Induced Tachy-Brady Syndrome: A patient taking medications like beta-blockers or antiarrhythmic drugs for other cardiovascular conditions may experience tachy-brady syndrome as a side effect of the medication. These medications can suppress the heart's normal electrical activity, leading to episodes of both rapid and slow heart rates.

4. Stimulant Abuse: Individuals who misuse stimulant drugs, such as cocaine or amphetamines, may experience tachy-brady syndrome as a result of the drug's effects on the heart's electrical system. These substances can disrupt the normal rhythm of the heart and cause alternating episodes of rapid and slow heart rates.

Diagnosis and Treatment:

Diagnosing tachy-brady syndrome involves a combination of medical history assessment, physical examination, electrocardiogram (ECG) readings, and sometimes additional tests like Holter monitoring or electrophysiological studies. Identifying the underlying cause is crucial for determining the most appropriate treatment approach.

Treatment options for tachy-brady syndrome may include:

1. Medications: Depending on the specific heart rhythm abnormalities and underlying conditions, medications may be prescribed to control tachycardia episodes, restore normal heart rhythm, and prevent bradycardia.

2. Pacemaker Implantation: In cases where bradycardia is the predominant issue, a pacemaker may be implanted. A pacemaker is a small device that helps regulate the heart's rhythm by sending electrical signals to stimulate the heart to beat at a consistent rate.

3. Ablation Therapy: In certain situations, catheter-based procedures like radiofrequency ablation may be performed to target and eliminate the abnormal electrical pathways causing tachy-brady syndrome.

4. Lifestyle Modifications: Making lifestyle changes, such as avoiding triggers like excessive caffeine or drug use, managing stress, and maintaining a healthy weight, can help minimize the frequency and severity of tachy-brady episodes.

Heart Blocks: Unveiling the Intricate Conduction System

Welcome to an exploration of heart blocks, a fascinating phenomenon within the heart's conduction system. In this comprehensive page, we will unravel the complexities of heart blocks, their types, causes, symptoms, and implications. Prepare to be amazed by the intricate workings of the heart's electrical pathways.

1. Understanding the Conduction System:

The heart's conduction system is responsible for coordinating its rhythm. It starts with the sinoatrial (SA) node, the natural pacemaker, and involves specialized pathways like the atrioventricular (AV) node and the bundle of His. These pathways ensure the synchronized contraction of the heart's chambers.

2. Heart Blocks: An Overview:

Heart blocks occur when electrical signals within the heart experience disruptions or delays. They are categorized into three types: first-degree, second-degree, and third-degree (complete) heart block.

3. Types of Heart Blocks:

a. First-Degree Heart Block:

This block involves a delay in electrical signal conduction, but all signals eventually reach the ventricles. It is often asymptomatic and considered a minor conduction abnormality.

b. Second-Degree Heart Block:

- Type I (Wenckebach): In this block, the PR interval progressively lengthens until a signal is blocked. It usually resolves on its own and has a favorable prognosis.

- Type II: Intermittent signals fail to reach the ventricles without a progressive PR interval lengthening. It carries a higher risk of progressing to a complete heart block.

c. Third-Degree (Complete) Heart Block:

No electrical signals pass from the atria to the ventricles. The ventricles establish their escape rhythm, which is typically slower. Immediate medical attention and pacemaker placement may be necessary.

4. Causes, Symptoms, and Implications:

Heart blocks can result from aging, heart diseases, medications, congenital heart defects, and cardiac surgeries. Symptoms vary but may include dizziness, fainting, fatigue, chest pain, and palpitations. Untreated heart blocks can lead to serious complications such as heart failure and sudden cardiac arrest.

5. Diagnosis and Treatment:

Diagnosis involves electrocardiogram (ECG/EKG) tests to evaluate the heart's electrical activity. Treatment options depend on the type and severity of the heart block and may include medication, lifestyle modifications, and pacemaker implantation for severe cases.

Conclusion:

Through this exploration of heart blocks, we've glimpsed the intricate conduction system of the heart. Understanding heart blocks and their implications is crucial for maintaining heart health. Remember, by unraveling the mysteries of the heart's electrical pathways, we can better appreciate the remarkable orchestration that keeps our hearts beating strong.

Unraveling the Mysteries of Bundle Branch Blocks: A Comprehensive Exploration

When a bundle branch block occurs in the setting of heart failure, it can further impair the heart's ability to pump effectively. This may lead to worsening symptoms of heart failure, such as fatigue, shortness of breath, fluid retention, and exercise intolerance. Managing heart failure in the presence of a bundle branch block typically involves a combination of medications, lifestyle modifications, and, in some cases, medical procedures or devices.

Bundle branch blocks occur due to disruptions in the electrical conduction system of the heart. The electrical signals that coordinate the contraction of the heart muscles are generated in the sinoatrial (SA) node, travel through the atria, and then pass through the atrioventricular (AV) node. From the AV node, the electrical impulses travel down specialized pathways called the bundle branches, which divide into the left bundle branch and the right bundle branch. These branches further divide into smaller branches, spreading the electrical signals to the ventricles.

Bundle branch blocks can happen for several reasons:

1. Structural Heart Disease: Conditions that affect the structure of the heart, such as coronary artery disease, heart attacks, cardiomyopathy, or heart valve abnormalities, can disrupt the normal conduction of electrical impulses through the bundle branches.

2. Aging: As people age, the electrical conduction system of the heart may undergo natural changes, leading to bundle branch blocks. The exact mechanisms behind age-related bundle branch blocks are not fully understood.

3. Cardiac Surgery or Procedures: Certain cardiac surgeries or procedures, such as coronary artery bypass grafting (CABG), heart valve surgery, or

catheter ablation, can damage or disrupt the bundle branches, resulting in bundle branch blocks.

4. Infiltrative Diseases: Some diseases, such as sarcoidosis or amyloidosis, can infiltrate the heart muscle and interfere with the normal conduction pathways, including the bundle branches.

5. Congenital Heart Defects: In some cases, bundle branch blocks can be present from birth due to congenital heart defects that affect the electrical conduction system.

In severe cases of bundle branch block, where there is a complete blockage of electrical impulses through the bundle branches, specialized treatment may be necessary. This can include the implantation of a pacemaker or cardiac resynchronization therapy (CRT). A pacemaker is a small device that is implanted under the skin and connected to the heart via wires. It helps regulate the heart's electrical activity by sending electrical impulses to stimulate the heart to beat at a normal rate. CRT is a type of pacemaker that specifically targets resynchronizing the contractions of the heart's ventricles, improving overall heart function.

Sinus Arrhythmia: Understanding, Management, and Real-Life Cases

Sinus arrhythmia is a common cardiac rhythm disorder characterized by irregular heart rate fluctuations during respiration. It is a physiological phenomenon that occurs due to the interplay between the respiratory and cardiovascular systems. While sinus arrhythmia is generally benign and does not require treatment, understanding its causes, identifying abnormal patterns, and managing associated symptoms can be crucial for individuals experiencing significant discomfort. This paper aims to explore the facts, solutions, and real-life cases related to sinus arrhythmia.

I. Facts about Sinus Arrhythmia:

1. Definition: Sinus arrhythmia refers to the irregularity in heart rate where the intervals between consecutive heartbeats vary with respiration.

2. Mechanism: Sinus arrhythmia is primarily caused by changes in vagal tone, resulting in variations in the firing rate of the sinoatrial (SA) node.

3. Respiratory influence: Sinus arrhythmia tends to be more pronounced during inspiration and less during expiration. This is due to the changes in intrathoracic pressure affecting vagal input to the heart.

4. Age-related changes: Sinus arrhythmia is more prominent in children and tends to decrease with age as the autonomic nervous system matures.

5. Association with health conditions: Sinus arrhythmia can be seen in individuals with normal cardiac function, but it may also occur in association with certain medical conditions such as heart disease, autonomic dysfunction, and respiratory disorders.

II. Clinical Presentation and Diagnosis:

1. Symptoms: Sinus arrhythmia is often asymptomatic and discovered incidentally. However, some individuals may experience palpitations, dizziness, or shortness of breath during pronounced irregularity.

2. Diagnosis: A diagnosis of sinus arrhythmia is usually made based on clinical evaluation, medical history, electrocardiogram (ECG) recordings, and analysis of heart rate variability (HRV).

III. Management and Treatment:

1. Reassurance: For most individuals with sinus arrhythmia, reassurance and education about the benign nature of the condition are sufficient, and no specific treatment is required.

2. Lifestyle modifications: Adopting a healthy lifestyle, including regular exercise, stress management techniques, and adequate sleep, can help regulate autonomic function and reduce the severity of sinus arrhythmia symptoms.

3. Treatment of underlying conditions: If sinus arrhythmia is associated with an underlying medical condition, such as heart disease or autonomic dysfunction, treating the primary cause may help alleviate the arrhythmia.

4. Medications: In rare cases where sinus arrhythmia causes significant symptoms or affects daily functioning, medication options such as beta-blockers or calcium channel blockers may be considered to regulate heart rate.

IV. Real-Life Cases:

1. Case 1: A 9-year-old child presented with palpitations during physical activity. After a thorough evaluation, it was determined that the child had sinus arrhythmia, which is common in children due to their developing autonomic nervous system. Reassurance and lifestyle modifications were recommended, leading to a resolution of symptoms.

2. Case 2: A middle-aged individual with a history of heart disease experienced pronounced irregular heartbeats during periods of stress. Further investigation revealed sinus arrhythmia associated with increased sympathetic activity. Treatment involved managing stress levels, optimizing cardiac function, and regular follow-up, resulting in improved symptoms and quality of life.

Atrial Fibrillation: Understanding and Real-Life Examples

Atrial fibrillation:

Atrial fibrillation (AF) is a prevalent cardiac arrhythmia characterized by irregular and rapid electrical signals in the atria, leading to poor blood flow. This page aims to provide a comprehensive overview of atrial fibrillation, highlighting its causes, symptoms, diagnosis, and real-life examples to enhance understanding and demonstrate the impact of this condition on individuals' lives.

Definition and Mechanism:

Atrial fibrillation occurs when the electrical signals in the heart's atria become chaotic, resulting in a rapid and irregular heartbeat. This disorganized electrical activity disrupts the normal coordination between the atria and ventricles, leading to compromised blood flow and potential complications.

Real-Life Example 1: Sarah's Journey

Sarah, a 55-year-old woman, experienced persistent fatigue, shortness of breath, and occasional palpitations during her daily activities. Concerned, she sought medical attention and was diagnosed with atrial fibrillation. Sarah's healthcare provider prescribed appropriate medications to manage her symptoms and reduce the risk of complications. Sarah's story serves as an example of how atrial fibrillation can significantly impact an individual's quality of life and the importance of seeking medical help for timely management.

Causes and Risk Factors:

Atrial fibrillation can have various causes, including underlying heart conditions such as hypertension, coronary artery disease, heart valve abnormalities, and heart failure. Other factors that contribute to AF include age, family history, obesity, excessive alcohol consumption, and certain chronic conditions like diabetes and thyroid disorders.

Real-Life Example 2: John's Experience

John, a 62-year-old man with a history of hypertension and diabetes, developed atrial fibrillation. Despite taking medication to manage his blood pressure and blood sugar, John's irregular heartbeat persisted. His healthcare provider recommended additional treatment options, including lifestyle modifications and anticoagulant medication to reduce his risk of stroke. John's case highlights the importance of addressing underlying risk factors and implementing a comprehensive treatment approach for individuals with atrial fibrillation.

Symptoms and Diagnosis:

The symptoms of atrial fibrillation can vary from person to person. Common symptoms include palpitations, rapid and irregular heartbeat, fatigue, shortness of breath, dizziness, and chest discomfort. Diagnosis typically involves a thorough medical history assessment, physical examination, and diagnostic tests such as electrocardiogram (ECG), echocardiogram, and Holter monitoring.

Real-Life Example 3: Emma's Journey

Emma, a 45-year-old woman, experienced occasional episodes of palpitations and shortness of breath. Concerned about her symptoms, she visited her healthcare provider who performed an ECG and diagnosed her with paroxysmal atrial fibrillation. Emma was advised to monitor her symptoms and keep a record to aid in the diagnosis and treatment planning. Emma's case emphasizes the importance of recognizing and documenting symptoms to facilitate accurate diagnosis and appropriate management of atrial fibrillation.

Treatment Options:

The treatment of atrial fibrillation aims to control heart rate, restore normal heart rhythm, and prevent complications such as stroke. Treatment options include medication, electrical cardioversion, catheter ablation, and lifestyle modifications.

Ventricular Fibrillation: Understanding and Real-Life Examples

Ventricular fibrillation is a life-threatening cardiac arrhythmia characterized by chaotic and irregular electrical activity in the heart's ventricles. It is a critical medical emergency that can lead to sudden cardiac arrest if not promptly treated. This page aims to provide a comprehensive overview of ventricular fibrillation, its causes, symptoms, diagnosis, and treatment options, accompanied by real-life examples to enhance understanding and illustrate the gravity of this condition.

Definition and Mechanism:

Ventricular fibrillation occurs when the heart's electrical signals become disorganized, resulting in the ventricles quivering ineffectively instead of pumping blood effectively throughout the body. This leads to a rapid decline in blood flow, causing loss of consciousness and potentially irreversible damage if not corrected promptly.

Real-Life Example 1: John's Story

John, a 52-year-old male, was enjoying a casual evening at home when he suddenly collapsed. His family immediately called emergency services, suspecting a heart attack. Paramedics arrived promptly and identified ventricular fibrillation as the cause of John's collapse. They initiated cardiopulmonary resuscitation (CPR) and used an automated external defibrillator (AED) to deliver an electric shock to his heart, successfully restoring a normal rhythm. John's experience highlights the critical importance of timely intervention in ventricular fibrillation cases.

Causes and Risk Factors:

Ventricular fibrillation can occur due to various factors, including coronary artery disease, heart attacks, heart failure, electrolyte imbalances, drug overdose, and genetic abnormalities. Additionally, certain risk factors may predispose individuals to ventricular fibrillation, such as a history of heart disease, previous heart attacks, family history of sudden cardiac death, and certain medications.

Real-Life Example 2: Lisa's Experience

Lisa, a 40-year-old woman with a history of heart disease, experienced a sudden onset of chest pain and shortness of breath while at work. Co-workers recognized the severity of her symptoms and immediately called emergency services. Paramedics arrived swiftly and diagnosed ventricular fibrillation. They promptly administered CPR and used an AED to restore her heart's normal rhythm. Lisa's case demonstrates the significance of recognizing symptoms and seeking immediate medical attention, especially for individuals with known risk factors.

Symptoms and Diagnosis:

The symptoms of ventricular fibrillation may include sudden loss of consciousness, absence of pulse, cessation of breathing, and pale or cyanosis (bluish skin.) Diagnosis is typically confirmed through an electrocardiogram (ECG) that reveals the characteristic irregular and chaotic waveform patterns associated with ventricular fibrillation.

Real-Life Example 3: Mark's Emergency

Mark, a 60-year-old man, was jogging in the park when he suddenly collapsed. A passerby witnessed the incident and immediately called emergency services. Paramedics arrived promptly, performed an ECG on site, and identified ventricular fibrillation as the cause. They initiated CPR and defibrillation, successfully restoring a normal heart rhythm. Mark's case highlights the importance of recognizing the symptoms of ventricular fibrillation and the critical role of early intervention in saving lives.

Treatment Options:

Immediate treatment of ventricular fibrillation involves cardiopulmonary resuscitation (CPR) and rapid defibrillation using an AED. Advanced cardiac life support (ACLS) interventions, including medications and electrical cardioversion, may also be employed in a hospital setting.

Ventricular Tachycardia: Racing Hearts and Life-Saving Interventions

Imagine a heart racing uncontrollably, beating faster than 100 times per minute. This is ventricular tachycardia (VT), a dangerous arrhythmia originating from the heart's ventricles. VT can be life-threatening if left untreated, making its recognition and prompt management crucial. In this paper, we will delve into the fascinating world of ventricular tachycardia, exploring its characteristics, how it is diagnosed, and the exciting treatment options available.

I. Unmasking Ventricular Tachycardia:

1. The Origin of Chaos: VT arises from abnormal electrical impulses originating in the ventricles, bypassing the heart's normal conduction pathways. This can occur due to various factors, such as scar tissue from previous heart attacks, structural heart disease, or inherited conditions affecting the heart's electrical system.

2. Decoding the ECG: By examining an electrocardiogram (ECG), a valuable diagnostic tool, we can identify VT through distinctive features. Look for wide QRS complexes (>0.12 seconds), a lack of preceding P waves, and a fast and regular or slightly irregular rhythm. The ECG's QRS morphology can also provide clues about the specific type and origin of VT.

3. Tales of Symptoms: VT can present with diverse symptoms, ranging from palpitations, dizziness, and fainting to more severe manifestations like chest pain and cardiac arrest. Understanding these varying symptoms can aid in early detection and intervention.

II. Unveiling the Diagnosis:

1. The ECG Detective: A 12-lead ECG is the initial step in diagnosing VT. It helps distinguish VT from other supraventricular tachycardias by revealing the unique QRS morphology, rate, and duration of the arrhythmia.

2. The Electrophysiological Enigma: Electrophysiological studies (EPS) may be conducted to delve deeper into the heart's electrical properties, pinpointing the specific site of VT origin. These studies involve the insertion of catheters into the heart to induce and map the arrhythmia, aiding in personalized treatment planning.

3. Seeking Clues in Images: Advanced imaging techniques, including echocardiography, cardiac magnetic resonance imaging (MRI), or coronary angiography, can help evaluate the heart's structure and identify any reversible causes of VT. These images provide valuable insights for targeted treatment approaches.

III. Battling Ventricular Tachycardia:

1. Swift Intervention: When VT causes hemodynamic instability or cardiac arrest, immediate electrical cardioversion is necessary. This dramatic technique involves delivering a synchronized electrical shock to reset the heart's rhythm and restore circulation.

2. Fighting the Storm: For stable VT, intravenous antiarrhythmic medications such as amiodarone, lidocaine, or procainamide may be administered to suppress the arrhythmia and restore normal sinus rhythm.

3. Guardians of the Heart: Long-term management of VT involves various approaches:

   a. Medicinal Warriors: Antiarrhythmic drugs like amiodarone, sotalol, or beta-blockers can be prescribed to prevent recurrent VT episodes. These medications aim to stabilize the heart's rhythm and reduce the risk of future arrhythmias.

b. Defenders Within Unleashing Life-Saving Power

When it comes to safeguarding lives, one technology stands out: the implantable cardioverter defibrillator (ICD). Designed for those at high risk of sudden cardiac death or recurrent ventricular tachycardia (VT), these tiny yet mighty devices are revolutionizing cardiac care. Implanted just beneath the skin, ICDs tirelessly monitor the heart's rhythm, ready to spring into action at a moment's notice. Armed with the ability to detect and correct dangerous arrhythmias through electric shocks, they serve as silent guardians, ensuring survival when every second counts. But that's not all – modern ICDs also offer additional perks like built-in pacemaker functionality and seamless data transmission to healthcare providers. With their power to both protect and improve lives, these defenders within are rewriting the rules of cardiac care, empowering patients to face each heartbeat with confidence.

Wolff Parkinson's White Syndrome: Unveiling Cardiac Pathway Marvels

Prepare to be captivated by the enigmatic world of Wolff Parkinson's White Syndrome (WPW).

In this concise page, we will explore the fascinating intricacies of this rare cardiac condition. Discover the extraordinary pathways within the heart that give rise to WPW, and unravel the mysteries behind its unique electrical circuitry.

1. Understanding WPW:

Wolf Parkinson's White Syndrome is a cardiac disorder characterized by an abnormal accessory pathway in the heart. This alternate pathway, known as the Bundle of Kent, creates irregular electrical circuits, leading to rapid and unpredictable heartbeats.

2. The Marvelous Pathways:

To grasp the essence of WPW, we must comprehend the heart's normal electrical system. The sinoatrial (SA) node, atrioventricular (AV) node, and bundle of His work together harmoniously to ensure synchronized contractions. However, in WPW, the presence of the accessory pathway disrupts this harmony, causing erratic electrical flow.

3. Implications and Symptoms:

WPW can result in episodes of rapid heartbeats called tachycardia. These episodes may occur suddenly, accompanied by palpitations, shortness of breath, dizziness, and chest discomfort. While WPW is generally benign, it can occasionally lead to life-threatening arrhythmias.

4. Diagnosis and Treatment:

Diagnostic techniques such as electrocardiogram (ECG/EKG) and electrophysiological studies help identify the characteristic "delta wave" on the ECG and locate the accessory pathway. Treatment options include medication to control heart rate and rhythm, catheter-based procedures like radiofrequency ablation to eliminate the accessory pathway, and, rarely, surgical interventions.:

Welcome to the captivating world of Wolf Parkinson's White Syndrome! Delving into the extraordinary pathways within the heart that contribute to this condition reveals a remarkable tale of cardiac electrical marvels. By unlocking the secrets of WPW, we gain a deeper appreciation for the intricate wonders that lie within our hearts.

Embracing the Beat of Resilience - The Holliday Heart Awakening

Introduction:

In a world where hearts beat to the rhythm of life, a unique phenomenon known as Holliday Heart emerges as a captivating enigma. We gather here today to embark on a journey of understanding, compassion, and empowerment. This manifesto is a call to arms, a testament to our collective commitment to unravel the mysteries of Holliday Heart and embrace the beat of resilience. Together, we shall shine a light on this intriguing condition, fostering awareness, support, and a newfound appreciation for the human heart's resilience in the face of adversity.

1. Unveiling the Heart's Party Animal:

Holliday Heart, named after its discoverer, Dr. Philip Holliday, is a condition characterized by an irregular heartbeat, specifically atrial fibrillation, that occurs following episodes of heavy alcohol consumption. It is as if the heart, known for its steadfast rhythm, temporarily succumbs to the allure of celebration. Yet, within this unconventional beat lies an opportunity for understanding and growth.

"Holiday heart" refers to a condition characterized by an irregular heart rhythm or arrhythmia that can occur after excessive alcohol consumption, particularly during holidays or weekends. It was first described in the late 1970s when a pattern was observed of individuals presenting with atrial fibrillation following heavy alcohol intake.

Here are some real-life cases, solutions, and an explanation of the condition:

Real-life cases:

1. Case 1: John, a 35-year-old male, experienced episodes of heart palpitations and rapid heartbeat after heavy alcohol consumption during a New Year's Eve celebration.

2. Case 2: Sarah, a 28-year-old female, developed atrial fibrillation after a night of heavy drinking at a bachelorette party.

Solutions:

1. Alcohol cessation: The primary solution for holiday heart is to avoid or limit alcohol consumption. For individuals experiencing holiday heart-related arrhythmias, it is recommended to abstain from alcohol to prevent recurrence.

2. Medical intervention: In some cases, medical intervention may be necessary to restore normal heart rhythm or manage the symptoms. Treatment options may include medications to control heart rate or rhythm, such as antiarrhythmic drugs or rate-controlling medications.

3. Lifestyle modifications: Adopting a healthier lifestyle, including regular exercise, a balanced diet, stress management techniques, and adequate sleep, can contribute to overall heart health and reduce the risk of arrhythmias.

4. Monitoring and follow-up: Regular monitoring by a healthcare professional is important to assess the heart's rhythm, make adjustments to medication if necessary, and ensure proper management of the condition.

Explanation of Holiday Heart:

Holiday heart is believed to be triggered by the direct effect of alcohol on the heart's electrical system. Excessive alcohol consumption can disrupt the normal electrical signaling pathways in the heart, leading to abnormal heart rhythms, such as atrial fibrillation or supraventricular tachycardia.

Alcohol is known to affect the autonomic nervous system, alter electrolyte levels, and cause dehydration, which can all contribute to the development of arrhythmias. The condition typically occurs in individuals without a history of heart disease or rhythm disorders, and the irregular heartbeat often resolves within a few days to weeks after alcohol cessation.

However, it's worth noting that holiday heart can also unmask underlying heart conditions or trigger arrhythmias in individuals with pre-existing cardiac abnormalities. Therefore, it is essential to seek medical evaluation and follow the recommended treatment plan to ensure appropriate management of the condition.

Unveiling the Hidden Link: Arteriosclerosis and the Spellbinding Dance of Heart Rhythms

Welcome to a world where the cardiovascular system reigns supreme, orchestrating the symphony of life within us. In this adventure, we unveil the secret relationship between arteriosclerosis—the hardening of arteries—and the mesmerizing dance of heart rhythms. Prepare to be captivated!

Clogged Pathways and Heart Flow:

Picture the arteries as the vital highways delivering life-sustaining blood to our organs. But what happens when arteriosclerosis strikes? These once-clear pathways become narrow and obstructed, disrupting the flow of blood. Hold on tight as we explore the impact on our heart's electrical beat.

Arteriosclerosis, also known as atherosclerosis, is a condition characterized by the buildup of plaque on the inner walls of arteries, leading to their narrowing and reduced blood flow. Arrhythmias, on the other hand, refer to abnormal heart rhythms. While arteriosclerosis and arrhythmias are distinct conditions, they can be linked in certain ways. Here are some correlations, risks, and potential solutions associated with arteriosclerosis and arrhythmias:

Correlations between Arteriosclerosis and Arrhythmias:
1. Ischemia: Arteriosclerosis can lead to reduced blood flow to the heart muscle, causing ischemia. Ischemia increases the risk of arrhythmias due to the disruption of normal electrical signaling in the heart.

2. Fibrosis: Arteriosclerosis-associated inflammation and damage to heart tissue can lead to fibrosis, the formation of scar tissue. Fibrosis can disrupt the electrical pathways in the heart, contributing to arrhythmias.

Risks Associated with Arteriosclerosis and Arrhythmias:
1. Heart Attack: Arteriosclerosis can lead to the formation of blood clots that can block blood flow to the heart, resulting in a heart attack. A heart attack can cause arrhythmias.

2. Stroke: Arteriosclerosis can also lead to the formation of blood clots that can block blood flow to the brain, causing a stroke. Stroke-related damage to the brain can increase the risk of arrhythmias.

3. Sudden Cardiac Arrest: Severe arrhythmias such as ventricular fibrillation can cause sudden cardiac arrest, a life-threatening condition. Arteriosclerosis can contribute to the development of arrhythmias that can trigger sudden cardiac arrest.

Solutions and Management:

1. Lifestyle Modifications: Adopting a heart-healthy lifestyle can reduce the risk of arteriosclerosis and arrhythmias. This includes maintaining a balanced diet, engaging in regular physical activity, avoiding tobacco use, managing stress, and controlling conditions like hypertension and diabetes.

2. Medications: Various medications can be prescribed to manage arteriosclerosis and arrhythmias. These may include antiplatelet agents, lipid-lowering drugs, blood pressure medications, and antiarrhythmic medications, among others. The specific medications prescribed depend on individual circumstances and should be discussed with a healthcare professional.

3. Medical Procedures: In some cases, medical procedures may be necessary to treat arteriosclerosis and arrhythmias. These can include procedures like angioplasty and stenting to open blocked arteries, coronary artery bypass grafting (CABG) to reroute blood flow around blocked arteries, or implantation of devices like pacemakers or implantable cardioverter-defibrillators (ICDs) to regulate heart rhythms.

The Elusive Connection: Unveiling the Relationship Between Diabetes and the Silent Arrhythmia

Introduction:
Diabetes mellitus, a chronic metabolic disorder characterized by impaired insulin function, affects millions of individuals worldwide. While diabetes is widely recognized for its impact on blood sugar regulation, there exists a lesser-known and intriguing association between diabetes and arrhythmias. Remarkably, diabetics can often be oblivious to the presence of arrhythmias, a phenomenon referred to as "silent arrhythmia." In this article, we delve into the reasons behind this intriguing connection, exploring the intricate relationship between diabetes and arrhythmias while shedding light on the mechanisms that underlie the lack of symptoms.

The Enigma of Silent Arrhythmia in Diabetics:
Silent arrhythmia refers to the absence of noticeable symptoms despite the presence of an irregular heart rhythm. This phenomenon is particularly prevalent in individuals with diabetes, posing a significant concern for both patients and healthcare providers. The reasons behind this elusive connection can be attributed to several interrelated factors:

1. Autonomic Neuropathy:
Diabetes can cause damage to the autonomic nervous system, leading to a condition known as autonomic neuropathy. This dysfunction affects the nerves responsible for regulating involuntary bodily functions, including heart rate and rhythm. As a result, the typical symptoms of arrhythmias are not conveyed to the diabetic individual, masking their awareness of the underlying cardiac irregularity.

2. Coexisting Cardiovascular Complications:
Diabetes is often accompanied by other cardiovascular complications, such as coronary artery disease, hypertension, and heart failure. These conditions can contribute to an altered perception of symptoms, as the diabetic patient's attention may be focused on managing these comorbidities, thereby overshadowing the presence of arrhythmias.

3. Silent Myocardial Ischemia:

Diabetics frequently experience silent myocardial ischemia, a condition characterized by reduced blood flow to the heart muscle without causing noticeable symptoms. This ischemia can disrupt the electrical conduction system of the heart, leading to arrhythmias. However, since the diabetic patient does not experience typical ischemic symptoms, such as chest pain or discomfort, the presence of arrhythmias may go unnoticed.

4. Glycemic Control:
Maintaining optimal glycemic control is crucial for individuals with diabetes. However, fluctuating blood glucose levels can influence the electrical stability of the heart, contributing to the development of arrhythmias. Paradoxically, the absence of symptoms may be attributed to the overall stability of blood glucose levels, which can diminish the risk of arrhythmias and subsequently render them "silent" in nature.

Conclusion:
The intricate relationship between diabetes and arrhythmias, particularly the phenomenon of silent arrhythmia, continues to baffle researchers and healthcare professionals alike. Autonomic neuropathy, coexisting cardiovascular complications, silent myocardial ischemia, and glycemic control intricacies are all important factors contributing to the lack of symptoms experienced by diabetic

Heart Blocks: An Electrifying Drama:

In the realm of cardiac electrophysiology, heart blocks represent a captivating tale of electrical conduction gone awry. The heart's electrical system, composed of the sinoatrial (SA) node, atrioventricular (AV) node, and specialized pathways, orchestrates the coordinated contraction of its chambers. Heart blocks occur when there is an interruption or delay in the electrical signals as they traverse this intricate network, leading to a disruption in the synchronized cardiac rhythm

First Act: The Sinister Sinus Node:
The sinus node, the heart's natural pacemaker, initiates the electrical impulses that set the rhythm for a healthy heartbeat. However, ischemia can infiltrate this critical protagonist, dampening its ability to generate regular electrical

signals. This results in sinus node dysfunction, causing a slow heart rate and paving the way for the emergence of heart blocks.

Second Act: The Atrioventricular (AV) Node's Dilemma:
As the electrical signals travel from the atria to the ventricles, they encounter the AV node, an essential relay station in the heart's electrical conduction system. Ischemia can disrupt the AV node, causing a delay or blockage of the electrical impulses. This captivating twist in the plot leads to different types of heart blocks, ranging from mild delays to complete blocks, each with its distinctive impact on cardiac function.

Third Act: Bundle Branch Blocks and Fascicular Blocks:
Intriguingly, ischemia can extend its reach to the specialized pathways known as the bundle branches and fascicles, further disrupting the normal flow of electrical signals. Bundle branch blocks and fascicular blocks manifest as delays or blockages in the transmission of electrical impulses, introducing a complex layer of intrigue to the narrative of heart blocks.

Climax: Ischemia's Legacy:
Ischemia's impact on heart blocks is not limited to the immediate disruption of electrical conduction. Prolonged ischemia can lead to irreversible damage to the heart muscle, impairing its ability to conduct electrical signals effectively. This legacy of ischemia can perpetuate the occurrence of heart blocks, creating a vicious cycle of electrical instability and compromised cardiac function.

Ischemia: A Stealthy Intruder:
Picture a bustling metropolis with its intricate network of roads. Ischemia, akin to a traffic jam, occurs when the heart muscle is deprived of an adequate supply of oxygen-rich blood. This deprivation arises from a narrowed or blocked coronary artery, often due to atherosclerosis or blood clot formation. The consequences of ischemia extend beyond the realm of simple oxygen deprivation, as they set the stage for the emergence of heart blocks, a captivating manifestation of electrical disruption.

Heart blocks refer to a disruption or delay in the electrical signals that regulate the heartbeat as they travel through the heart's conduction system. This can cause an abnormal rhythm or a slower heart rate. There are different types of heart blocks, including first-degree, second-degree, and third-degree heart blocks. Here's a simplified explanation of each type:

1. First-Degree Heart Block: In first-degree heart block, there is a delay in the electrical signals as they pass through the conduction system. However, all signals eventually reach the lower chambers of the heart (ventricles). It is usually not a cause for concern and may not require treatment.

2. Second-Degree Heart Block: Second-degree heart block is further classified into two types: Type 1 (Wenckebach) and Type 2 (Mobitz II).

   - Type 1 (Wenckebach): In Type 1 second-degree heart block, there is a progressive lengthening of the delay between the electrical signals, leading to the occasional failure to transmit a signal to the ventricles. This results in a skipped heartbeat or a dropped beat.

   - Type 2 (Mobitz II): In Type 2 second-degree heart block, there is a consistent and sudden blockage of some electrical signals, causing occasional dropped beats without any pattern. This type of heart block may be more concerning and require medical attention.

3. Third-Degree (Complete) Heart Block: In third-degree heart block, also known as complete heart block, there is a complete blockage of the electrical signals between the upper chambers (atria) and the lower chambers (ventricles) of the heart. As a result, the atria and ventricles beat independently, and the ventricles may have a slower and less regular rhythm. Third-degree heart block often requires medical intervention, such as the placement of a pacemaker, to restore a normal heart rate and rhythm.

It's important to note that heartblocks can vary in severity and symptoms. Some individuals with heart blocks may not experience any noticeable symptoms, while others may experience dizziness, fainting, fatigue, or chest discomfort. The diagnosis and management of heartblocks are typically done by healthcare professionals, such as cardiologists or electrophysiologists, who assess the individual's specific condition and determine the most appropriate treatment plan.

This simplified explanation provides a general overview of heart blocks, but it's always best to consult with a healthcare professional for a comprehensive evaluation and personalized guidance based on your specific situation.

Unraveling the Mysteries: Extra Pathways in Babies and the Puzzling World of Arrhythmias.

The mystery of extra pathways in pediatrics; In some newborns and young children, there can be additional electrical pathways in the heart that are not typically present in healthy individuals. These pathways, known as accessory pathways, can develop during fetal development and persist after birth. They create abnormal electrical connections between the atria and the ventricles, bypassing the normal conduction pathway.

The most well-known accessory pathway is called the bundle of Kent, which forms an abnormal connection between the atria and the ventricles. The development of accessory pathways during fetal development can have significant consequences for the individual's heart function and overall health. These extra pathways create abnormal electrical connections between the atria and the ventricles, bypassing the normal conduction pathway and altering the heart's electrical conduction system.

`One of the most significant consequences of accessory pathways is the potential to cause rapid heart rates or arrhythmias. In individuals with accessory pathways, such as the bundle of Kent in Wolff-Parkinson-White (WPW) syndrome, electrical signals can travel through both the normal conduction pathway (AV node) and the accessory pathway simultaneously. This creates a short circuit in the heart's electrical system, leading to the development of a specific type of arrhythmia called supraventricular tachycardia (SVT).

During SVT episodes, electrical signals can rapidly loop between the atria and ventricles through the accessory pathway, resulting in an abnormally fast heart rate. This can lead to symptoms such as palpitations, rapid heartbeat, dizziness, shortness of breath, and in severe cases, fainting or cardiac arrest. The rapid heart rate during SVT can also affect the heart's pumping efficiency, potentially compromising blood circulation to vital organs.

Additionally, accessory pathways can increase the risk of other arrhythmias and complications. The abnormal electrical connections may disrupt the coordinated contraction of the heart chambers, leading to irregular heart rhythms such as atrial fibrillation (AF) or ventricular arrhythmias. These arrhythmias can further impair the heart's ability to pump blood effectively, potentially resulting in symptoms like fatigue, chest discomfort, and even heart failure.

Moreover, individuals with accessory pathways are at an increased risk of developing complications related to SVT, such as the development of blood clots within the heart. SVT episodes can cause turbulence in the atria, favoring the formation of blood clots. If a blood clot dislodges and travels to other parts of the body, it can cause a stroke or other life-threatening complications.

Due to these potential consequences, early detection and appropriate management of accessory pathways in babies and individuals are crucial. Diagnosis typically involves a combination of medical history assessment, physical examination, electrocardiography (ECG), and potentially further cardiac tests like electrophysiological studies. Treatment options may include medications to control heart rate and rhythm, catheter-based procedures to ablate or eliminate the accessory pathway, or in certain cases, surgical interventions.

In summary, the presence of accessory pathways that develop during fetal development can lead to significant consequences, primarily related to the development of abnormal heart rhythms and associated symptoms. Timely diagnosis and appropriate management are vital to minimize the risk of complications and ensure the well-being of individuals with accessory pathways.

The presence of accessory pathways in babies can be puzzling, as it may not always cause symptoms or be immediately apparent. However, in some cases, babies with accessory pathways may experience palpitations, rapid heartbeat, or even more severe symptoms such as fainting or cardiac arrest. Prompt diagnosis and appropriate management are crucial to ensure the well-being of these infants.

The Duel of Hearts: Pacemakers vs. Implantable Cardioverter Defibrillators (ICDs)

In the realm of cardiac devices, two titans stand tall—the pacemaker and the implantable cardioverter defibrillator (ICD). These remarkable technologies have revolutionized the management of heart rhythm disorders, captivating the medical world and transforming the lives of countless individuals. Join us on an intense journey as we delve into the duel of hearts, exploring the similarities, differences, and captivating capabilities of pacemakers and ICDs. Brace yourself for an exhilarating showdown that will keep you hooked until the final beat.

Round 1: The Rhythm Regulators

In this round, we witness the battle of rhythm regulation. Pacemakers take center stage as they deliver electrical impulses to maintain a steady heart rate, combating bradycardia and ensuring a harmonious cardiac rhythm. On the other hand, ICDs unleash their power in detecting and terminating life-threatening arrhythmias, protecting against sudden cardiac death. Prepare to be enthralled as we explore the unique mechanisms through which these devices restore and preserve the heart's rhythm; detecting life-threatening arrhythmias.

Round 2: Tailored Solutions

In this round, we delve into the personalized nature of these devices. Pacemakers, designed with various programmable features, offer tailored solutions to meet individual patients' unique needs. From rate modulation to activity sensing, these devices adapt to the ever-changing demands of the heart. Conversely, ICDs provide a multi-dimensional defense strategy, with customizable settings to detect and treat specific arrhythmias. Discover the art of customization as we explore how these devices adapt to safeguard each patient's cardiac well-being.

Final Round: Beyond the Duel

As the duel concludes, we take a step back to appreciate the collective impact of pacemakers and ICDs on the lives of those they serve. These devices have become symbols of hope, granting individuals a new lease on life and empowering them to pursue their dreams. Witness the awe-inspiring stories of resilience and triumph that showcase the profound influence of these devices beyond the confines of the duel.

The clash between pacemakers and ICDs has mesmerized the world of cardiac care, captivating both medical professionals and patients alike. From rhythm regulation to life-saving interventions, these devices have rewritten the narrative of heart health. As we bid farewell to the duel, we are left with a profound appreciation for the transformative power of pacemakers and ICDs. Their legacy of saving lives and restoring rhythm resonates, reminding us of the indomitable spirit of the human heart.

Cardioversion: Restoring Heart Rhythm with Electric Precision

Introduction:

In the world of cardiac treatments, there's a remarkable procedure called cardioversion that holds the power to restore normal heart rhythm. By using controlled electric shocks, cardioversion acts like a symphony conductor, bringing order to chaotic heartbeats. This has the potential to make a significant difference in people's lives. This captivating process, with its careful timing and precision, offers hope to those struggling with irregular heartbeats.

When irregular heartbeats or arrhythmias disrupt the normal rhythm of the heart and pose a significant risk to an individual's health, medical professionals may turn to a powerful intervention known as cardioversion. This procedure aims to restore the heart's normal rhythm and improve its function.

Cardioversion involves the delivery of a carefully controlled electric shock to the heart. The shock is administered through specialized equipment, such as a defibrillator or cardioverter, which delivers a precisely timed electrical current to the heart. The electrical shock essentially resets the heart's electrical system, allowing it to resume its regular rhythm.

The decision to perform cardioversion is based on the type and severity of the arrhythmia, as well as the individual's overall health and medical history. Cardioversion is commonly used for two types of arrhythmias: atrial fibrillation (AF) and certain types of ventricular arrhythmias.

In atrial fibrillation, the atria of the heart fibrillate or quiver instead of contracting effectively. This leads to an irregular and often rapid heartbeat. Cardioversion can be performed in cases of persistent or long-standing atrial fibrillation, where medications or other treatments have not successfully restored a normal rhythm. By delivering a controlled electrical shock to the heart, cardioversion helps to synchronize the atrial electrical signals and restore a regular heartbeat.

Certain ventricular arrhythmias, such as ventricular tachycardia (VT) or ventricular fibrillation (VF), may also necessitate cardioversion. VT is characterized by a rapid heartbeat originating from the ventricles, while VF is a life-threatening arrhythmia where the ventricles quiver instead of contracting effectively. In these cases, cardioversion is utilized as an emergency procedure to quickly restore normal heart rhythm and prevent sudden cardiac death. Immediate intervention and defibrillation are crucial in such critical situations.

Cardioversion is typically performed in a controlled medical environment, such as a hospital or specialized cardiac care unit. Before the procedure, the individual may receive sedation or anesthesia to ensure their comfort and minimize any potential discomfort during the shock delivery. The healthcare team carefully monitors the individual's vital signs throughout the procedure to ensure their safety.

It is important to note that cardioversion is not a permanent solution for arrhythmias. While it can successfully restore the heart's normal rhythm, underlying factors contributing to the arrhythmia, such as heart disease or certain medical conditions, may need to be addressed to prevent future recurrences. Medications, lifestyle modifications, and further interventions, such as catheter ablation or implantable devices like pacemakers or implantable cardioverter-defibrillators (ICDs), may be recommended as part of a comprehensive treatment plan.

The powerful intervention of cardioversion is employed when irregular heartbeats or arrhythmias bring power to the heart's normal rhythm.

By delivering a precisely controlled electrical shock, cardioversion can restore the heart's regular rhythm and improve its function. This procedure is a valuable tool in managing certain arrhythmias and mitigating the associated risks to an individual's health.

Idiopathic Arrhythmias: A Call to Unwavering Focus

Introduction:

Idiopathic arrhythmias, characterized by abnormal heart rhythms of unknown origin, pose a significant challenge to medical professionals and patients alike. These elusive conditions have the potential to disrupt lives, yet they often receive less attention and research compared to other well-known cardiac disorders. This manifesto is to emphasize the importance of maintaining focus on idiopathic arrhythmias, highlighting the need for increased awareness, research, and support for those affected by these conditions.

1. The Prevalence and Impact of Idiopathic Arrhythmias:

Idiopathic arrhythmias are more common than one might think. An idiopathic arrhythmia may develop due to a collection of excitable cells in the heart that cause it to beat in an abnormal rhythm these conditions can occur in individuals of any age and can lead to serious consequences, including fainting, heart failure, and sudden cardiac arrest...

By understanding the prevalence and potential risks associated with idiopathic arrhythmias, we can appreciate the urgent need for focused attention.

2. The Diagnostic Challenge:

The lack of a clear underlying cause makes diagnosing idiopathic arrhythmias a complex task. Often, patients undergo a battery of tests and evaluations, enduring a prolonged period of uncertainty and anxiety. The absence of a definitive diagnosis can be frustrating for both patients and medical professionals, leading to a diminished focus on these conditions. However, we must recognize that persistent focus and concerted efforts are essential for unraveling the mysteries surrounding idiopathic arrhythmias.

The ECGs of idiopathic outflow tract VAs are characterized by positive R waves in all inferior leads and deep S waves in both leads aVR and aVL.

3. Patient Empowerment and Support:

Individuals living with idiopathic arrhythmias often face physical, emotional, and psychological burdens. The lack of a clear cause or cure can leave them feeling helpless and isolated. In such cases, it becomes crucial to provide a strong support system that empowers patients to actively manage their condition. By creating patient-centered initiatives, support groups, and educational resources, we can foster resilience and ensure that patients do not lose focus in their journey toward better health.

Maintaining an unwavering focus on idiopathic arrhythmias is crucial for advancing our understanding and improving the lives of those affected. By recognizing the prevalence and impact of these conditions, prioritizing research, providing patient support, and promoting collaboration, we can ensure that idiopathic arrhythmias receive the attention they deserve.

Unveiling the Intriguing World of Arrhythmias: Unraveling the Rhythmic Mysteries of Stress Testing

During a stress test, the individual undergoes physical exercise, usually on a treadmill or stationary bike, to increase the heart rate and evaluate how the heart responds to the stress. The stress test aims to assess the heart's function, blood flow, and identify any abnormalities or symptoms that may arise during exercise.

Some common arrhythmias triggered by the stress tests are;

Premature Ventricular Contractions (PVCs): The Unexpected Heartbeats

Amid the heart's symphony, a rogue drummer emerges, introducing a captivating twist to the rhythm. Premature ventricular contractions (PVCs) disrupt the harmonious beat, injecting unexpected accents into the cardiovascular performance. These early, abnormal electrical impulses originating from the ventricles create an intriguing syncopation that demands attention. While often harmless, frequent or symptomatic PVCs raise the curtain on potential underlying heart conditions, urging us to explore the untold stories hidden within the arrhythmic tapestry

Premature Ventricular Contractions (PVCs):

- Description: PVCs are extra heartbeats originating from the ventricles.

- Symptoms: Often none, but may cause palpitations or skipped beats.

- Stress Test Findings: Stress testing can evaluate the frequency and response of PVCs during exercise.

Supraventricular Tachycardia (SVT): Prepare for an electrifying spectacle as the atria take the lead in a dance of rapid rhythms. Supraventricular tachycardia (SVT) sets the stage ablaze, showcasing a variety of captivating moves, including atrial fibrillation, atrial flutter, and paroxysmal supraventricular tachycardia. These spellbinding performances, induced by exercise, unveil the intricate pathways and triggers that govern the heart's electric choreography. Witnessing SVT during stress testing offers a window into the heart's secrets, guiding us toward tailored treatments and a deeper understanding of these mesmerizing arrhythmic phenomena.

Supraventricular Tachycardia (SVT):

- Description: SVT encompasses various arrhythmias arising above the ventricles.

- Symptoms: Rapid heartbeat, palpitations, lightheadedness, chest discomfort.

- Stress Test Findings: Stress testing can help diagnose SVT and evaluate its response to exercise.

Exercise-Induced Atrial Fibrillation (AF):

Atrial fibrillation (AF) is a common type of arrhythmia characterized by rapid and irregular electrical activity in the atria, the upper chambers of the heart. While AF is typically diagnosed through symptoms and electrocardiogram (ECG) recordings, it may also be evaluated during a stress test.

In the case of atrial fibrillation, the stress test can help determine if exercise triggers or exacerbates AF. The individual's heart rate, rhythm, blood pressure, and ECG are continuously monitored during the stress test to assess any changes or abnormalities.

If atrial fibrillation occurs or is induced during the stress test, it may suggest several possibilities:

1. Exercise-induced AF: Some individuals may experience AF specifically during exercise or physical exertion, which is known as exercise-induced AF. This can provide valuable information about the triggers and nature of AF in that individual.

2. Underlying AF: In individuals who have a history of AF or suspected AF but may not be experiencing symptoms at the time of the stress test, exercise can sometimes reveal the presence of underlying AF.

Detecting AF during a stress test can guide treatment decisions and management strategies. It can help healthcare professionals determine appropriate interventions, such as medication adjustments, rate control strategies, or further diagnostic tests.

Atrial Fibrillation (AF):
   - Description: AF is the most common type of arrhythmia, characterized by irregular and rapid contractions of the atria.
   - Symptoms: Palpitations, shortness of breath, fatigue, dizziness, chest discomfort.
   - Stress Test Findings: AF may be induced or exacerbated during stress testing, leading to an irregular heart rate response.

Bradycardia

During a stress test, *bradycardia* refers to a condition where the heart rate slows down significantly or becomes abnormally low during exercise or physical stress. Normally, during exercise, the heart rate increases to meet the increased demand for oxygen and nutrients by the body. However, in some cases, the heart rate may not increase appropriately, or it may even decrease, resulting in bradycardia during a stress test.

Bradyarrhythmias (abnormally slow heart rhythms) can occur due to various factors, including:

1. Sinus Node Dysfunction: The sinus node, often referred to as the heart's natural pacemaker, may not function properly, leading to a slower heart rate.

2. Medications: Certain medications, such as beta-blockers or calcium channel blockers, can lower heart rate and cause bradycardia.

3. Hypothyroidism: An underactive thyroid gland can affect the heart's electrical conduction system, leading to bradycardia.

4. Vagal Stimulation: Stimulation of the vagus nerve, which can occur during exercise or due to other factors, can slow down the heart rate.

5. Athlete's Heart: Well-trained athletes may have a naturally slower resting heart rate, which can persist during exercise and cause bradycardia during a stress test.

It's important to note that not all cases of bradycardia during a stress test are problematic or indicative of an underlying health issue. In some cases, it may be a normal physiological response, particularly in individuals who are highly fit or have well-conditioned hearts.

.

Bradycardia:
 - Description: Bradycardia refers to an abnormally slow heart rate.

- Symptoms: Fatigue, dizziness, fainting, shortness of breath.

- Stress Test Findings: Stress testing can assess heart rate response during exercise and uncover exercise-induced bradycardia.

Long QT Syndrome (LQTS)

In the context of a stress test, *Long QT Syndrome (LQTS)* refers to a genetic disorder affecting the heart's electrical system that can be evaluated or assessed during the test. LQTS is characterized by abnormal prolongation of the QT interval on an electrocardiogram (ECG), which represents the time taken for the heart's electrical signals to repolarize.

During a stress test, the individual's heart rate, blood pressure, and ECG are continuously monitored. The QT interval is measured at rest and may also be monitored during exercise. This assessment helps evaluate the response of the QT interval to physical stress or exercise. Individuals suspected of having LQTS may undergo a stress test to observe any exercise-induced changes in the QT interval. If there are significant changes in the QT interval or the development of arrhythmias during exercise, it may indicate an increased risk for adverse cardiac events in individuals with LQTS

The stress test in LQTS aims to assess the risk of exercise-induced arrhythmias, such as Torsades de Pointes, which is a potentially life-threatening ventricular arrhythmia associated with LQTS. Exercise can sometimes trigger arrhythmias in individuals with LQTS due to the increased demand on the heart and changes in the electrical conduction system...

Long QT Syndrome (LQTS):

- Description: LQTS is a genetic disorder affecting the heart's electrical system, leading to abnormal QT intervals on an electrocardiogram (ECG).

- Symptoms: Fainting, arrhythmias, sudden cardiac arrest.

- Stress Test Findings: Stress testing can help assess exercise-induced arrhythmias and QT interval changes in individuals suspected of having LQTS.

In conclusion, stress testing is a valuable diagnostic tool in the field of cardiology that provides important insights into the heart's response to physical exertion. This non-invasive procedure helps healthcare professionals assess the presence of underlying heart conditions, evaluate exercise tolerance, and guide treatment decisions.

The information obtained from stress testing can aid in the diagnosis of conditions such as coronary artery disease, heart valve disorders, and heart rhythm abnormalities. It can help determine the severity of the condition, assess the effectiveness of ongoing treatment, and guide decisions regarding further diagnostic procedures or interventions.

The Rhythm's Rebellion: Unraveling Medication-Induced Arrhythmias

Introduction:

Medication-induced arrhythmias, a captivating phenomenon within the realm of cardiology, occur when certain medications disrupt the heart's normal rhythm and electrical conduction. While medications play a crucial role in treating various medical conditions, they can occasionally lead to unintended consequences, including disturbances in the heart's electrical activity. This captivating chapter unravels the intricacies of medication-induced arrhythmias, exploring the mechanisms, risk factors, and management strategies associated with this fascinating phenomenon.

Mechanisms:

Medication-induced arrhythmias can stem from various mechanisms, each with its unique impact on the heart's electrical system. Some medications alter the heart's electrical signals by affecting ion channels responsible for the conduction of electrical impulses. For instance, certain medications may prolong the QT interval, a segment of the electrocardiogram (ECG) that reflects the time it takes for the heart to repolarize. Prolongation of the QT interval can increase the risk of a specific arrhythmia called torsades de pointes, a potentially life-threatening form of ventricular tachycardia.

Other medications may interfere with the normal functioning of the atrioventricular (AV) node, which regulates the conduction of electrical impulses between the atria and ventricles. This interference can lead to abnormalities in heart rhythm, such as heart block or AV nodal reentrant tachycardia.

Risk Factors:

Several factors contribute to an individual's susceptibility to medication-induced arrhythmias. Certain medications have a higher propensity to cause rhythm disturbances, especially those that directly affect the heart's electrical properties. Furthermore, individual characteristics, such as underlying heart disease, electrolyte imbalances, genetic predispositions, and the presence of other medications, can increase the risk of developing medication-induced arrhythmias. It is essential for healthcare professionals to carefully consider these factors when prescribing medications and monitor patients for any potential adverse effects.

The management of medication-induced arrhythmias involves a multidimensional approach aimed at balancing the benefits of the medication with the potential risks to the heart's rhythm. The primary goal is to ensure the individual's safety while providing effective treatment for the underlying medical condition.

Medication-induced arrhythmias occur when certain medications affect the electrical signals that regulate the heartbeat. Here are some examples of medications and their potential effects on the heart's rhythm:

A. Antibiotics: Certain antibiotics, such as macrolides (e.g., erythromycin, azithromycin), fluoroquinolones (e.g., ciprofloxacin), and some antifungal medications (e.g., ketoconazole) can prolong the QT interval in the heart's electrical cycle. Prolonged QT intervals can lead to a specific type of arrhythmia known as torsades de pointes, which can be life-threatening.

B. Antidepressants: Some antidepressant medications, particularly those in the class of selective serotonin reuptake inhibitors (SSRIs), tricyclic antidepressants (TCAs), and certain monoamine oxidase inhibitors (MAOIs), can also prolong the QT interval. This effect increases the risk of developing arrhythmias, including torsades de pointes.

C. Antiarrhythmics: Ironically, certain medications used to treat arrhythmias themselves can cause arrhythmias as a side effect. Some antiarrhythmic drugs, such as class IA drugs like quinidine and disopyramide, and class III drugs like amiodarone and sotalol, have the potential to disrupt the heart's normal rhythm if not used appropriately.

Cases of medication-induced arrhythmias and potential solutions:

Case 1: Jane, a 55-year-old woman with hypertension, developed bradycardia (slow heart rate) after starting a new blood pressure medication.

Solution: In this case, the solution may involve discontinuing or adjusting the dosage of the medication that is causing the bradycardia. The healthcare provider may prescribe an alternative medication or lower the dosage of the current medication to avoid further slowing of the heart rate.

Case 2: Mark, a 40-year-old man with a history of arrhythmias, experienced ventricular fibrillation (a life-threatening arrhythmia) after taking a specific antibiotic medication.

Solution: In this case, immediate medical intervention is required. Mark should seek emergency medical care to receive appropriate treatment for ventricular fibrillation, such as defibrillation to restore a normal heart rhythm. After stabilization, the healthcare provider will discontinue the medication that triggered the arrhythmia and may explore alternative antibiotics that have a lower risk of causing arrhythmias.

Case 3: Sarah, a 65-year-old woman with a history of heart failure, developed atrial fibrillation after starting a new medication for another medical condition.

Solution: In this case, the healthcare provider may prescribe antiarrhythmic medications to help control and stabilize Sarah's heart rhythm. They will closely monitor her response to the medication and adjust the dosage or switch to alternative medications if needed. Additionally, managing Sarah's underlying heart failure through appropriate medications and lifestyle modifications may also help improve her overall heart health and reduce the risk of arrhythmias.

Case 4: David, a 50-year-old man with a history of depression, developed prolonged QT interval (a potentially dangerous arrhythmia) after starting a new antidepressant medication.

Solution: The solution in this case may involve discontinuing the antidepressant medication and consulting with a psychiatrist or healthcare provider to explore alternative medications that have a lower risk of prolonging the QT interval. It is important to prioritize the individual's mental health needs while considering the potential risks associated with certain medications.

The Enigmatic Scheme: Anxiety Feigning as Arrhythmias

In the realm of cardiovascular health, a captivating and wicked intrigue unfolds as anxiety assumes the role of a villain, cunningly disguising itself as arrhythmias. With calculated precision and anxiety, the mastermind behind this malevolent charade ensnares both patients and medical professionals in its intricate web of deception. Let us venture into this shadowed landscape, where anxiety, the devious antagonist, commonly masquerades as arrhythmias, orchestrating its sinister scheme.

Anxiety, a formidable adversary lurking within the corridors of the mind, derives pleasure from instilling fear, worry, and apprehension. Yet, its malevolence extends beyond the realm of thoughts, infiltrating the very fabric of the body. When anxiety seizes control, it sets in motion a cascade of physiological responses, priming the body for an imagined threat. The heart, an unwitting accomplice, succumbs to anxiety's manipulation, racing and pounding to mirror the erratic rhythms of true arrhythmias.

Arrhythmias, the authentic antagonists within the realm of cardiac pathology, disrupt the harmonious synchrony of the heart's electrical system. They unleash chaos, compelling the heart to beat irregularly, either too rapidly or too slowly, akin to a malevolent puppeteer pulling the strings. Palpitations skipped beats, and a sense of impending doom marked their presence, casting victims into a state of unease and vulnerability.

Yet, anxiety, the treacherous impersonator, adeptly mimics the symptoms of arrhythmias, casting an ominous veil of doubt and confusion upon the scene. The accelerated heartbeat, the constricting grip around the chest, the breath held captive by invisible forces—these are the weapons of anxiety's artful deception. Cloaked in its malevolent guise, anxiety effortlessly assumes the identity of arrhythmias, leading both patients and medical professionals astray in their quest for truth.

Anxiety feigning as arrhythmias refers to a situation where a person's anxiety or panic attack symptoms mimic the symptoms of an irregular heartbeat or abnormal heart rhythm, known as arrhythmias. In other words, the individual may experience physical sensations in their chest that feel like a racing heart, skipped beats, or palpitations, which are typical signs of arrhythmias. However, these symptoms are not caused by any underlying heart condition but rather by the person's heightened anxiety or panic response.

Anxiety is a natural response to stress or perceived threats, and it can manifest in various physical and psychological symptoms. When a person experiences intense anxiety or a panic attack, their body goes into a "fight-or-flight" mode, triggering a surge of stress hormones such as adrenaline. This can lead to increased heart rate, elevated blood pressure, and other physiological changes that mimic the symptoms of arrhythmias.

It's important to note that anxiety feigning as arrhythmias does not mean that the person is intentionally faking or pretending to have a heart condition. Instead, it indicates that the symptoms they are experiencing are a result of their anxiety rather than a primary cardiac issue. These symptoms can be distressing and alarming for the individual, as they may genuinely believe that there is something wrong with their heart.

If someone is experiencing anxiety feigning as arrhythmias, it's essential for them to seek medical evaluation to rule out any potential underlying heart conditions. A healthcare professional can perform a thorough examination, which may include tests such as an electrocardiogram (ECG) or a Holter monitor to monitor the heart's electrical activity over a specific period. These tests can help determine whether the symptoms are due to anxiety or an actual arrhythmia.

Treatment for anxiety feigning as arrhythmias typically involves addressing the underlying anxiety or panic disorder. This may include a combination of therapies such as cognitive-behavioral therapy (CBT), medication, stress management techniques, and lifestyle modifications. By managing and reducing anxiety levels, the symptoms that mimic arrhythmias can often be alleviated.

With meticulous scrutiny, these healthcare heroes employ electrocardiograms, Holter monitors, and event recorders as their investigative instruments, capturing the heart's electrical symphony. They strive to separate fact from fiction, to expose the true nature of the villain masquerading within. By delving into psychological assessments and engaging in open dialogue with patients, they glean additional insights, illuminating anxiety's sinister presence.

Education and awareness stand as potent weapons against this duplicitous adversary. Empowering patients with knowledge, helping them comprehend the insidious nature of anxiety and its capacity to masquerade as arrhythmias, becomes a crucial step toward victory. Open lines of communication between patients and medical professionals become vital conduits for the exchange of fears, experiences, and suspicions, aiding in the ultimate unmasking of the true villain.

Treatment diverges, for anxiety and arrhythmias are distinct foes, each requiring a tailored approach. Anxiety calls for the implementation of relaxation techniques, therapeutic interventions, and, when necessary, pharmacological support to dismantle its menacing grip. True arrhythmias, on the other hand, necessitate a specialized armamentarium.

In conclusion,

The intricate workings of the heart's electrical conduction system, along with the presence of bundle branch blocks and accessory pathways, can be likened to the harmonious collaboration of musicians in an orchestra. The conductor, represented by the conduction system, orchestrates the rhythm and coordination of the heart's contractions.

Just as each musician in an orchestra plays a crucial role, the bundle branches and accessory pathways serve as key performers in transmitting electrical signals throughout the heart. However, when these pathways encounter disruptions, such as bundle branch blocks or abnormal accessory pathways, the heart's rhythm can become discordant, leading to cardiac arrhythmias.

Similar to a discordant note in a musical piece, arrhythmias disrupt the heart's natural rhythm and require intervention. The treatment journey, guided by healthcare professionals, parallels the conductor's role in correcting the discordant note and restoring harmony. Through various approaches like medication, lifestyle modifications, or procedures such as pacemaker implantation or catheter ablation, the aim is to restore the heart's rhythm and ensure optimal cardiac function.

Just as an orchestra's success hinges on the collaboration and synchronization of all musicians, the successful management of cardiac arrhythmias relies on the collaboration between patients, healthcare professionals, and specialists. By working together harmoniously, tailored treatment plans can be created, leading to improved outcomes and enhanced quality of life for those experiencing cardiac arrhythmias.

In this book, we have explored the complexities of bundle branch blocks, accessory pathways, and the management of cardiac arrhythmias. By drawing parallels to the symphony of an orchestra, we hope to provide a unique perspective that aids in understanding these conditions and emphasizes the importance of collaboration, skilled intervention, and the pursuit of harmony in the intricate rhythm of the heart.

May this book serve as a valuable resource and guide in navigating the world of cardiac arrhythmias, empowering individuals, healthcare professionals, and researchers alike to continue striving for optimal cardiac health, where the heart's symphony plays with perfect rhythm and harmony.